Grow Green

Contents

INTRODUCTION

A HEALTHY DIET FOR LIFE

Well-planned plant-based diets can support healthy lifestyles at every age, from pre-parenthood, through pregnancy and breast-feeding, childhood and adulthood, and on into later years.

THE IMPORTANCE OF GOOD NUTRITION

Your diet during pregnancy and that of your infant during the first year of life can affect your child's health 40,50 or even 60 years later. It is therefore of utmost importance that during pregnancy you and your baby are provided with good nutrition. During pregnancy you will require extra nutrition to support your growing fetus and to allow for changes in your body.

GAINING SUPPORT

If you do not live in a supportive environment may you may receive criticism of your vegan diet and lifestyle. Pediatricians and dietitians may raise doubts about adequacy of the vegan diet and in some cases advise against it. These recommendations are usually the result of misinformation, and by sticking to your vegan principles and following the simple guidelines in this book, you can ensure that your child thrives.

GUIDELINES

Many theories abound on the feeding and raising of children, and healthcare professionals may make recommendations which differ from guidelines set out in this book in general, a more relaxed attitude to weaning and feeding children is currently in vogue. However, it is important to bear in mind that this book is only a guide, and should not be used as a substitute for medical care in the event of any possible health problems.

WHAT IS VEGANISM
INTRO TO YOUR NEW LIFESTYLE

Veganism is a philosophy and way of living which seeks to exclude—as far as is possible and practicable—all forms of exploitation of, and cruelty to, animals for food, clothing or any other purpose; and by extension, promotes the development and use of animal-free alternatives for the benefit of humans, animals and the environment. In dietary terms it denotes the practice of dispensing with all products derived wholly or partly from animals.

WHAT DO VEGANS EAT

A great deal - you'll soon find a whole new world of exciting foods and flavors opening up to you. A vegan diet is richly diverse and comprises all kinds of fruits, vegetables, nuts, grains, seeds, beans and pulses - all of which can be prepared in endless combinations that will ensure you're never bored. From curry to cake, pasties to pizzas, all your favorite things can be suitable for a vegan diet if they're made with plant-based ingredients

CHAPTER 1
PRE-CONCEPTUAL NUTRITION

Women may wait for a positive pregnancy test to improve their diet, stop drinking alcoholic beverages, and generally opt for more positive habits. While adopting a healthy lifestyle at any stage of pregnancy is beneficial, research suggests that a mom's habits before conception also influence her baby's well-being at birth and for his or her entire lifetime. Priming the body for pregnancy optimizes both a mom's health and that of her child.

MEN'S HEALTH

Little is mentioned of men's health before conception, but this is also important. A man is producing sperm all the time, and sperm takes 70 days to develop. Therefore the state of their health may affect the quality and quantity of the sperm.

WOMEN'S HEALTH

It is accepted that women should take care of her health before pregnancy, and nutritional status is important in a relation to pregnant outcome. The developing fetus is most susceptible to nutrition deficiency the first trimester (first three months). However, a well-balanced vegan diet will not leave you short of any nutrients needed to prepare for a healthy pregnancy. As in all stages of life, the importance of ensuring an intake of a reliable source of b12 and of vitamin d at this time

It is recommended that in addition to eating foods rich in folic acid, women considering pregnancy should take a folic acid supplement each day before pregnancy and for 12 weeks during pregnancy. Although a vegan diet is generally rich in folic acid, it is highly recommended that intake is increased. Folic acid is a b vitamin, and it can help to prevent spina bifida and other conditions in which the brain or spinal cord does not develop properly. Folic acid is found in green leafy vegetables, fortified breakfast cereals, wholemeal bread , pulses(beans, peas and lentils) and yeast extract.

PREGNANCY PLANS

Preconception care involves more than a single visit to the gynecologist, internal medicine physician, certified nurse midwife, or nurse practitioner in the months prior to a pregnancy. Priming the body for pregnancy is an ongoing pursuit that ideally begins early in a woman's reproductive life.

Pregnancy preparedness makes sense, particularly because many pregnancies are unexpected. A developing fetus is highly susceptible to birth defects and other problems during the first eight weeks of pregnancy, a time when women may not realize they are expecting and typically long before their first visit with a healthcare professional to address their pregnancy.

Preconception care should be tailored to meet a woman's needs, accounting for chronic conditions such as overweight or underweight, type 1 or type 2 diabetes, and hypertension. Women who have had a pregnancy end in a low birth weight baby (less than 51/2 pounds), a preterm infant (born between the 20th and 37th week of gestation), a child with a birth defect, or infant death should seek medical advice prior to conceiving to prevent problems with subsequent pregnancies

CHAPTER 2
PREGNANCY – FIRST FEW MONTHS

Pregnancy can lead to changes in many of your daily routines and habits, including what you eat and how much exercise you get. But most of all: women's bodies change during pregnancy so their unborn children get enough nourishment and other things they need. These changes already start happening in early pregnancy, and become more and more noticeable as time goes on. Women gain more weight towards the end of pregnancy than they do in the early months. This is not only due to the weight of the growing baby. Much of the weight gained is extra fluid (water) in the body. This is needed for things like the baby's circulation, the placenta and the amniotic fluid.

EATING FOR TWO

Recommendations for many vitamins and minerals are higher during pregnancy, but as a physiological response to pregnancy the absorption of many nutrients is increased. The majority of pregnant women (including vegans) can meet these increased needs by consuming a varied diet. Just follow your appetite and avoid excesses or under-over eating.

A pregnant woman's weight alone is not a good indicator of how well her baby is doing – not even of how fast her baby is growing. This depends on a lot of factors. It is not possible to say for sure how much the baby will weigh at the end of pregnancy. Ultrasound scans and other tests can only give us a rough idea of how the baby is developing and how much he or she might weigh at birth.

Recommended Weight Gain

Whilst recommendations for many vitamins and minerals are higher during pregnancy, the increase in energy(calorie) requirements is relatively small. General guidelines include a little weight gain of approximately 1-2 kg (2-4 ln) during first trimester, and in the second and third trimesters a weight gain of 5kg per semester is common. There is little, if any, increase in calorific needs during the first and second trimesters. However, in order to support the recommended weight gain during the third trimester an extra 200 calories per day will be required. 200 calories is a fairly small increase, but it is important to consume these extra calories wisely. You should, for example, increase the intake of fresh fruit and vegetables and/or wholemeal bread and hummus, instead of drinking a can of coke and eating a bar of chocolate ! the coke and chocolate will provide the calories, but not the vital nutrients required for the health of the woman and her growing baby.

Three meals a day should be eaten, starting with breakfast. Although breakfast may not be terribly appealing if you are suffering from morning sickness, it is an important meal as it comes after a long period without food. It is important to provide regular supply of nutrients to the growing fetus. Babies do not do well if they fast for hours on end.

THE BODY MASS INDEX (BMI)

The body mass index (BMI) is the most common way to determine whether people are underweight, overweight or have a normal weight. It is a measure of the relationship between weight and height. A BMI under 18.5 is considered to be underweight, a BMI between 18.5 and 25 is "normal weight," and a BMI between 25 and 30 is "overweight." If someone has a BMI over 30 they are considered to be very overweight (obese).

BMI alone is not enough to say whether someone's weight is likely to cause health problems, though. Many overweight people are very healthy. It can become more of a problem if they have particular illnesses too, such has type 2 diabetes. Having a BMI above 30 is likely to increase the risk of related health problems.

WHAT DO GUIDELINES RECOMMEND

Recommendations about BMI and weight gain in pregnancy are as follows:

For women who were underweight before becoming pregnant (women with a BMI below 18.5 to be "underweight"): recommended weight gain of between 12.5 and 18 kilograms during pregnancy.
For women who had a normal weight before becoming pregnant (women with a BMI between 18.5 and 24.9 to have a "normal weight"): recommended weight gain of between 11.5 and 16 kilograms during pregnancy.
For women who were overweight before becoming pregnant (women with a BMI between 25 and 29.9 to be "overweight"): recommended weight gain of between 7 and 11.5 kilograms during pregnancy.
For women who were obese before becoming pregnant (women with a BMI over 30 to be "obese"): recommended weight gain of between 5 and 9 kilograms during pregnancy.

Problems with weight gain

If weight gain is slow or non-existent, more food is required. Food should be eaten more often. The types of food eaten should be higher in calories and lower in fiber. If weight gain is high, then sweet or fatty food should be replaced with fresh fruit, vegetables, pulses and grains (wholemeal bread and pasta). If the diet is already fairly healthy, then more exercise should be taken on a daily basis, e.g. walking, swimming, etc.

If you are suffering from nausea during the early stages of pregnancy you may find that your appetite is reduced, in which case weight gain can initially be quite slow. However this should not be of concern and an increase in appetite later on in pregnancy will more than make up for any lapses.

Can putting on too much or too little weight be a problem

Women who gain a lot of weight in pregnancy have a higher risk of certain health problems and complications during childbirth. For instance, they are more likely to have a very big child with a birth weight of over 4,000 g or 4,500 g (macrosomia), and are more likely to need a Cesarean section. They are also more likely to have difficulties losing the extra weight after giving birth.

On the other hand, if a woman does not gain enough weight and is undernourished in pregnancy, it can harm her growing baby: babies are then often born too early (preterm birth) or often weigh too little at birth.

CHAPTER 3
KEY NUTRIENTS FOR PREGNANCY

FOLIC ACID

Ensure adequate folic acid, folate or folacin consumption to protect against neutral tube defects such as spina bifida. Studies suggest this is plentiful in the diets of vegan adults. However, women considering having a baby and those who are pregnant should take a folate supplement as well as consuming foods rich in the vitamins. All women wishing to conceive should take 400mcg(0.4mg) per day and continue this during the first 12 weeks of pregnancy. Pregnant women should take 300mg per day.

VITAMIN B12

Pregnant women do not require more than the average 3ug per day from fortified foods (or 10ug/day if relying on supplements). During pregnancy your own laid down body stores of b12 are not readily available to the fetus, which builds up its own supply from your daily intake of the vitamins. If B12 intake is low during pregnancy, the fetus will not have adequate stores of the vitamin and this may lead to a deficiency sometime after birth, even though you may have no clinical symptoms. A supplement should be taken if fortified foods are not consumed on a regular basis.

CALCIUM

Your body will need more calcium during pregnancy. Vegan diets being rich in fruit and vegetables and free of animal protein help conserve calcium. If you struggle to get enough calcium from green leafy vegetables and fortified foods (e.g. fortified milks, yogurts, etc.), take a supplement to ensure calcium requirements are met. Additionally, it is possible to purchase calcium carbonate powder which can be mixed into food or added to home-made bread.

IRON

There is an extra demand for iron for the developing baby and to form hemoglobin. Women who had heavy periods or were slimming before pregnancy may start their pregnancy with low iron stores, and can end up tired and anemic. An adequate intake of iron rich foods should be consumed, and foods which contain a lot of vitamin c should be eaten with the meal, such as a glass of fruit juice or a piece of fruit, as this aids the absorption of iron. Tea can reduce the absorption of iron, so either intake should be reduced, tea drunk only between meals. It is not wise to take iron tablets unless prescribed, because too much iron can interfere with the absorption of other minerals and can cause constipation.

ZINC

There is evidence from the general population that malformations occurring in some infants may be linked to zinc insufficiency in their mothers. Human milk is not a rich source of this mineral, and during breastfeeding infants draw on their body reserves laid down during the last three months of pregnancy. Thus premature babies may be at risk of zinc deficiency. Intakes of zinc by adult vegans are similar to those of omnivores, and there is no recommended increase during pregnancy. Ensure a mixture of zinc-rich food such as nuts, seeds, beans and cereals, or sprouting zinc-rich beans and seeds.

FLUID

Drink plenty of fluids during pregnancy. The state of pregnancy is a «watery» one and you will require extra water for making additional blood for yourself, your body, and the 6 to 12 pints of amniotic fluid in your uterus. At least six to eight (200ml) glasses per day should be consumed, preferably in the form of water, fruit juice or vegetable juice. The balance of water needed can be obtained from the watery fruits, vegetables, soups and salads which are abundant in the vegan diet.

CHAPTER 4
VEGAN PROTEINS

Proteins are known as the building blocks of life: In the body, they break down into amino acids that promote cell growth and repair. (They also take longer to digest than carbohydrates, helping you feel fuller for longer and on fewer calories—a plus for anyone trying to lose weight.) You probably know that animal products—meat, eggs and dairy—are good sources of protein; unfortunately, they can also be high in saturated fat and cholesterol. What you may not know is that you don't need to eat meat or cheese to get enough protein.

In the next few pages you'll find your personal diary of plant based protein sources that will help you build your healthy lifestyle.

GREEN PEAS

Foods in the legume family are good sources of vegetarian protein, and peas are no exception: One cup contains 7.9 grams—about the same as a cup of milk.

QUINOA

quinoa is unique in that it contains more than 8 grams per cup, including all nine essential amino acids that the body needs for growth and repair, but cannot produce on its own. (Because of that, it's often referred to as a "perfect protein.") Plus, it's amazingly versatile: Quinoa can be added to soup or vegetarian chili during winter months, served with brown sugar and fruit as a hot breakfast cereal, or tossed with vegetables and a vinaigrette to make a refreshing summer salad

NUTS

All nuts contain both healthy fats and protein, making them a valuable part of a plant-based diet. But because they are high in calories—almonds, cashews, and pistachios for example, all contain 160 calories and 5 or 6 grams of protein per ounce—choose varieties that are raw or dry roasted

BEANS

There are many different varieties of beans—black, white, pinto, heirloom, etc.—but one thing they all have in common is their high amounts of protein. Two cups of kidney beans, for example, contain about 26 grams (almost the same as a Big Mac, which has 25 grams!).

CHICKPEAS

Also known as garbanzo beans, these legumes can be tossed into salads, fried and salted as a crispy snack, or pureed into a hummus. They contain 7.3 grams of protein in just half a cup, and are also high in fiber and low in calories.

TEMPEH AND TOFU

Foods made from soybeans are some of the highest vegetarian sources of protein: Tempeh and tofu, for example, contain about 15 and 20 grams per half cup, respectively. They're highly nutritious, and they can really take on the taste and texture of whatever type of food you're looking for.

EDAMAME

Not crazy about meat substitutes? Get your servings of soy the way it appears in nature: Straight from the soybean, still in the pod. Boiled edamame, which contains 8.4 grams of protein per half cup, can be served hot or cold and sprinkled with salt. Try it as a snack, an appetizer before dinner, or added to salads or pastas

LEAFY GREENS

Vegetables don't have nearly as much protein as legumes and nuts,, but some do contain significant amounts—along with lots of antioxidants and heart-healthy fiber. Two cups of raw spinach, for example, contain 2.1 grams of protein, and one cup of chopped broccoli contains 8.1 grams.

HEMP

you can find it in some cereals and trail mixes, or you can buy hemp seeds (10 grams of protein in 3 tablespoons) and add them to smoothies, pestos, or baked goods. Hemp milk can also be a dairy-free way to add protein to your diet, and it's even lower in calories than skim milk.

AVOCADO

Avocadoes provide all 18 essential amino acids necessary for the body to form a complete protein. Unlike the protein in steak, which is difficult for most people to digest, avocado protein is readily absorbed by the body because avocadoes also contain fiber.

Chia seeds

These seeds are an easy way to add protein (4.7 grams per ounce, about two tablespoons) and fiber to almost any recipe: Chia seeds can be sprinkled over salads, stirred into yogurt or oatmeal, blended into smoothies, or they can take center stage: They plump up and take on a gelatinous texture when soaked in a liquid, forming a rich and creamy pudding-like treat.

Sesame, sunflower and poppy seeds

Don't discount the other seeds in your pantry, either; the more familiar varieties are also high in protein and healthy fats. (Per volume, sunflower seed kernels contain the most protein—7.3 grams per quarter cup—followed by sesame seeds and poppy seeds at 5.4 grams each.)

Seitan

Another meat substitute popular with vegetarians, seitan is made from wheat gluten, seasoned with salt and savory flavors and loaded with protein—36 grams per half cup, more than either tofu or tempeh. It looks like duck meat and tastes like chicken, and can be used in any recipe that calls for poultry.

Non-dairy milk

Milk alternatives aren't just for the lactose intolerant: (Plain soy milk, for example, contains about 100 calories per cup.) Soy milk has the most protein, at 4 to 8 grams per 8 ounces, but almond, hemp, and rice milk also contain about 1 gram per cup.

Cocoa powder

Bet you didn't know you can get protein from chocolate! Unsweetened cocoa powder—the type used in baking or making hot chocolate from scratch—contains about 1 gram of protein per tablespoon.

CHAPTER 5
SUGGESTED MEAL PLAN DURING PREGNANCY

BREAKFAST

-wholemeal toast spread with vegan margarine and marmite (or yeast extract) or peanut butter- or both!
-porridge and dried fruit with nut topping
-muesli and fresh fruit with fortified soya milk
-scrambled tofu with chopped onion and peppers on toast
-crispbreads spread with margarine and nut butter
-baked beans and lightly-fried mushrooms on wholemeal toast

SNACKS

-fresh and dried fruit
-nuts
-fruit smoothies (made with liquidized soft fruit and/or vegetables and fortified soya milk)
-wholemeal crackers and vegetable patè
-yogurt (fortified vegan versions)

LUNCH

-vegan spread or hard cheese, pickle and salad sandwich
-veggie burger, wholemeal bun, lettuce, tomatoes, beansprouts,. fresh green salad with French dressing.
-vegetable bean soup and baked potato
-samosas or onion bhajis with salad
-fruit cake

DINNER

-starter: vegetable soup and/or green salad
-main courses: vegan versions of lasagna, spaghetti Bolognese, shepherd's pie, stew, curry, vegetable briani, quiche, etc.

DESSERT

-Fresh fruit salad and ice-cream
-Fruit crumble and custard made with fortified soya milk
-Apple pie and soya crème
-Cake (fruit, vanilla sponge, chocolate, fudge, carob)
-Tofu cheesecake

BEVERAGES

-Pure water
-Fruit juices
-Fortified soya milk shakes
-Coffee/tea
-Herbal teas/infuses

Note: large amount of caffeine have in some cases been associated with various problems in pregnancy. Caffeine is a stimulant and crosses the placenta. It appears in the fetus's blood in the same concentration as in the mother's blood. It is advised that pregnant women should moderate their caffeine intake to no more than 300md/day, which is equivalent to approximately four cups of coffee per day.

CHAPTER 6
COPING WITH COMMON FOOD-RELATED PREGNANCY PROBLEMS : ADVICE TO PREGNANT WOMEN

MORNING SICKNESS :

-Many women find eating little is the best remedy. Eat five or six small meals per day, and try to eat something every few hours because you may feel sick when you're really hungry.

-Avoid greasy or fried foods, as these take longer to digest. If the smell of cooking makes you queasy, ask someone else to cook while you are out of the house, or try eating cold foods like sandwiched, cereal, soya yogurt, nut/seed butters and crackers, or fruit.

-Don't lie down directly after eating; sit for at least 15 minutes after eating.

-Keep a snack such as crackers or dry cereal by the bed, and eat a little on waking up in the night of before getting up in the morning.

-Try making mixtures like mashed potatoes and chopped vegetables, or vegetables and rice, because starchy foods are often more appealing than vegetables.

-Foods containing ginger have been found to relieve nausea for some women

-Try peppermint tea

Heartburn and indigestion

-Try small frequent meals
-Eat slowly
-Drink liquids between meals rather than with them
-Stay upright after eating
-Do not go to bed on a full stomach
-If it's worse at night, a slightly tilted bed or propped pillows can help
-Avoid spicy and acid foods, and fizzy drinks

Constipation

-Ensure an adequate intake of fiber rich foods
-Drink plenty of fluids
-Take gentle exercises

CHAPTER 7
BREAST-FEEDING AND FORMULA MILKS

BREAST IS BEST

The first food for a vegan baby should ideally be breast milk. Breast-fed infants of well-nourished vegan women grow and develop normally. Infants receives many benefits from breast-feeding, including immune system enhancement, protection against infection, and reduced risk of allergies. Moreover, as human breast milk is the natural food for baby humans, it is also probably contains substances needed by growing infants which may not even be known to be essential and which are not included in infant formulas. Nursing mothers derive benefits such as reduced risk of premenopausal breast cancer, release of stress-relieving hormones, and sheer convenience. For all these reasons, breastfeeding is strongly encouraged.

INFANT FORMULAS

Unfortunately there is currently no infant formula available which is suitable for vegans. There are soya formulas on the market, but these are not 100% vegan as they are fortified with vitamin D3, which is made from lanolin (a grease produced by sheep's skin and extracted from their wool).

SOYA FORMULA AND SOYA MILK

Some concern has been expressed regarding the relationship between the glucose content of soya formula and tooth decay in children. Glucose syrup has several properties that make its use in soya formulas appropriate: it is easily absorbed and utilized by infants even when the gut mucosa is damaged, and the use of glucose syrup as the carbohydrate in a soya formula ensures a similar osmolality to breast milk.

It is easily mixed with water, which is essential for home preparation, and the naturally bitter taste of soya protein is effectively masked by glucose syrup without causing undue sweetness.

Note :Formula should be fed from a feeding bottle. However, between the ages of 6 and 12 months a beaker or cup should increasingly be used. The use of a bottle should not be prolonged, and teeth should be cleaned after feeds. Regarding tooth decay, evidence indicates that the quantity of sugar eaten is less important than the time taken to consume it and the interval before further sugar is eaten. If sugary foods or drinks are consumed, it is better to ensure they are finished relatively quickly rather than eaten over several hours, as the mouth pH can be restored within 30 minutes.

The Diet for Breastfeeding

The diet for breastfeeding is similar to that recommended for pregnancy although calories, protein and vitamin B12 are higher.

- The recommended calorie intake is 500 calories above the usual intake.
- Consume a B12 supplement (10mcg per day) or ensure a regular source of foods fortified with vitamin B12 (4mcg per day)
- Protein requirements are 11g above the usual intake from the birth of your baby until 6 months of age, and from the age of 6 months it can be reduced to 6g above the usual intake.
- Take a supplement of 260mg of folic acid per day
- Current recommendations for calcium consumption are 1250mg per day for breast-feeding women.
- A good intake of vitamin D via sun exposure or (in the winter) vitamin D fortified products (or supplements) all year round.
- Good calcium intake should be ensured
- No extra iron is need for breast-feeding women.

If your diet contains little or no vitamin B12 you will produce milk with very low levels of vitamin B12 as this vitamin Is Important for the developing nervous system, it is crucial that your infant has a reliable source. If your diet does not contain a reliable daily source of vitamin b12, your child should receive a daily source of vitamin B12 such as a B12 droplet. The vitamin D content of breast milk may vary with diet and sun exposure.

Readers may also have heard of docosahexaenoic acid or DHA, a fatty acid which appears to be important for eye and brain development, and is found primarily in animal foods. However, vegans can make DHA form another fatty acid called alpha-linolenic acid, which will be contained in the breast milk if your diet includes good sources such as flaxseed oil, ground flaxseed, and rapeseed oil. Reducing the use of other oils such as corn oil, sunflower oil and safflower oil, and limiting foods containing hydrogenated fats, will also help your breast-fed infant make more DHA. These oils contain linoleic acid, and hydrogenated fats contain trans-fatty acids which interfere with DHA production.

WEIGHT LOSS AND MILK LOSS

After birth, body weight is probably about 7lb (3.5kg) over the weight before pregnancy. This is the body store needed for breast-feeding. It is important not to try and lose this weight by dieting as it may not be possible to get enough energy and nutrients for you and your baby. If too little food is eaten while breast-feeding then quantities of milk produced are liable to be lower. These extra pounds are usually shred gradually during breast-feeding because of a loss of calories in breast milk.
Small frequent meals are best. Extra fluid is required at this time so the opportunity should be takes to have nutritious drinks like fruit and vegetable juices, fortified soya milks, soups and smoothies, which will provide extra calories as well.
It makes sense to continue breast-feeding for a year, if possible, because breast milk is such a rich source of nutrients.

CHAPTER 8
BRINGING UP YOUR BABY

BIRTH – 6 MONTHS

From birth to 6 months all of your baby's nutritional needs can be met through breast milk. If your baby is also receiving bottle feeds, you will make less breast milk. The more your baby breast-feeds, the more milk you will produce. Feeding frequency should be as with breast-feeding-on demand. Left to themselves, bottle-fed babies consume little more than breast-fed babies and are only slightly heavier.

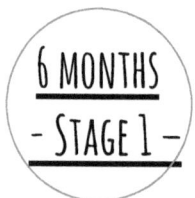

6 MONTHS
- STAGE 1 –

Note that all infants have a high requirement for vitamin D to enable calcium deposition in bone. It is encouraged that vitamin drops containing vitamin A, C and D be used for all children from 6 months to 5 years of age, weather vegan, vegetarian or omnivore. Some vitamin drops contain no animal products and are suitable for vegans.

At 6 months solid foods can be introduced, but the weaning process should not be hurried if your baby is content with breast milk alone. Pay attention to the signals your baby gives out. Breast-feeding should be continued (alongside the introduction of solids) for as long as is comfortable for both you and your baby.

Solids should not be introduced into the diet before age of four months, do not be pressurized to introduce solids before this time. This is because your baby's body systems, physiology and development, are not ready for solids and can only cope with breast milk or formula milk.

The best time to introduce solid foods to your baby is just before breast-or bottle-feeding. Starting solids is a very gradual process, so be patient and go slowly. The classic "first food" is mashed banana, which is very digestible, sweet and a good introduction to foods. Other popular first foods are apples, pears, peaches, and vegetables such as carrots, potatoes, and spinach (which are cooked and then mashed or pureed and sieved), and baby rice.

The first few weeks are merely an introduction, and you should not be tempted to try to fill your baby up with solids. When they have had enough babies will turn away their head, clamp their mouth shut or spit the food out! Offer one type of food only and observe how well it is tolerated, then wait two to three days before trying another food. This gives your baby's digestive system time to get used to each new food before the introduction of additional ones. If two or more foods are introduced at the same time and your baby has diarrhea, colic or other digestive problems, it will be difficult to identify the culprit. Start with around 1-2 tsp of food and gradually increase up to 6 tsp. how much is fed to your baby depends entirely on how much they will eat. A rough guide might be a quarter of a very ripe mushy banana for a few days (or for a week), and the following week another soft fruit such as apple sauce. The foods during this first stage should be bland with smooth consistency.

If your baby is not interested in the first few times solids are introduced, it is advised to try again in another week. When your baby is ready they will let you know. Your baby might be hungry at any time od the day or night. Babies cannot tell the time but they know what they need. Prepare cooked vegetables plainly.

Do not add salt, sugar or spices. Good introductory vegetables are parsnips, sweet potatoes, yams and carrots. Still start feeds with breast or bottle, but now very gradually increase the amount of solid food given afterwards. Solids should only be given by spoon or hand, and never added to a bottle or feed.

TYPICAL FEED FOR ONE DAY AT STAGE 1

1st feed- breast or bottle

2nd feed- breast or bottle

3rd feed- 1 tsp baby rice mixed with 1tbsp milk from feed or 1-2 tsp unsweetened fruit puree

4th feed- breast or bottle

5th feed- breast or bottle

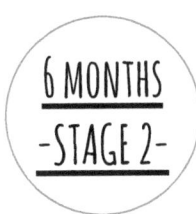

Try and move gradually from solid food at one feed in the day to solid food at two and then three feeds. Follow your baby's appetite and move at their pace.

Avoid all baby foods that contain sugar or artificial sweeteners. Sugar contains no vitamins, minerals or protein, and can lead to obesity, both now and later in the child's life. Sweetened foods also confuse and seduce the appetite, tending to satisfy hunger quickly and displace healthful foods. Do not add salt to foods.

TYPICAL FEED FOR ONE DAY AT STAGE 2

1st feed- breast or bottle

2nd feed- breast or bottle followed by 1-2 tsp baby rice mixed with 1tbsp milk from feed or 1-2 tsp unsweetened fruit puree

3rd feed- breast or bottle milk followed by 1-2 tsp vegetable puree or 1-2 tsp pureed fruit

4th feed- breast or bottle followed by 1-2 pureed fruit

5th feed- breast or bottle

6-7 MONTHS

At 6 months of age, wheat, corn and oat-based cereals can be introduced. Use well-cooked wholegrain cereals which must be mushy in consistency. If your family has a history of wheat, soya or corn allergies, start with rice or oat cereals. A small amount of mashed banana or breast milk can be added to the cooked cereal for easy introduction.

By 6 months of age, iron stores in omnivorous, vegetarian and vegan infants will become depleted, and it is important that iron-rich foods are included in the diet. Iron-fortified infant cereals are a good way to supply iron to begin infants. To enhance iron absorption, add a source of vitamin C such as green leafy vegetables, citrus fruits, blackcurrant or orange juice to the meal. Foods containing generous amounts protein such as mashed cooked pulses, mashed tofu and soya yogurt are generally introduced at around 7-8 months of age.

8-10 MONTHS

From 8-10 months of age gradually adjust your baby's feeds to fit in with the rest of the family's meal times. Your baby should be used to a spoon and experimenting with foods that has soft lumps or is mashed, e.g mashed potato. Bake potatoes whole to preserve vitamins and mash, with a small amount of water or breast milk. Try mashing them with cooked beetroot to make them pink, something that delights babies of this age. Your baby will be ready for fresh fruits, e.g. pears, peaches, plums and melons. Try finger foods such as toast or rusks.

Never leave your baby alone whilst eating or drinking, they could easily choke whilst you back is turned. Avoid giving chunks or sticks of vegetables to children under 3 years of age because of the danger of choking.

Your baby may also be taking a drink from a cup, suitable drinks (in addition to bottle or breast9 include cooled boiled water or diluted fruit juice, e.g. apple, watermelon, pear, peach and prune. Children's teeth are at most risk from tooth decay. Babies should never be left with sugar drinks or juices in feeding bottles or reservoir feeders.

TYPICAL FEED FOR ONE DAY AT 8-10 MONTHS

On waking- breast or bottle or unsweetened fruit juice or cooked boiled water
Breakfast- stewed or fresh fruit, baby rice or breakfast cereal, toast fingers with margarine/yeast extract, breast or bottle
Lunch- cooked vegetables puree with protein
Snack- mashed or fruit puree or a piece or finger food fruit with breast or bottle milk
Dinner- breast or bottle milk

10-12 MONTHS

At 10-12 months the texture of foods can be chopped, finely grated or blended. Your baby is likely to be holding a spoon and trying to feed on their own. They should be receiving a variety of vegetables, and after a tolerance to various foods is established, they can be offered blended salads. Try blending avocado, tofu, apple sauce and cooked greens with nut butters. The introduction of peanuts and nuts to the diet of infants from allergic families should be delayed until three years old of age or at an age advises by their medical practitioner. For infants from families with no known allergy there is no need to specifically delay the introduction of peanuts.

During this time period well-cooked whole grains (e.g. stained rice, barley and oatmeal) as well as high protein cereals (e.g. soya beans and wheat germ) may be introduced. Your infant should be eating a wide variety of vegetables now, including spinach and cabbage, along with root vegetables and fruits

12+ MONTHS

From 12 months of age infants can share the same meals as the rest of the family, with additional snacks in-between. Add legumes (peas and beans) to the menu, but be sure all beans are cooked until quite soft, and that the skins (especially soya) are removed. A thin split-pea soup is a good introduction to legume protein. Check stools to see whether the beans are being digested well. If the stool smells sour, if your baby's bottom becomes reddened or irritated, or if parts of beans are seen, wait a while before trying legumes again. Some infants do not tolerate whole legumes until two or three years of age. However other soy products (such as oy milk and tofu) and grains will meet the child's nutritional needs.

Hummus, made with chickpeas and tahini (sesame seed butter), is a tasty protein and calcium rich-food. Another winner is avocado, rich in riboflavin, essential fatty acids, potassium and copper. Small pieces of ripe avocado can be eaten as finger food, or blended with water or fruit juice. Smooth nut and seed butters spread on bread or crackers are another good finger food. It is now a good time to introduce bread to the diet. Start with toast, as it is easier for your infant to chew. Don't forget how much children, even young ones, love noodles. Pastas, enriched with artichoke or other vegetable flours and served with gravies and sauces, provide energy and protein.

 Also try to get your infant at this age to enjoy raw vegetables such as carrots and cucumbers. Grate vegetables finely, or try putting a dab of peanut butter, tahini or almond butter on vegetables to entice the infant to eat. Plain tofu and rice cakes are other healthful snacks.

 As solid foods become a larger part of the diet, be sure to give foods which provide concentrated sources of calories and nutrients such as mashed firm tofu, bean spreads, mashed avocado and cooked dried fruits. Frequent meals and snacks help ensure adequate energy intakes. The fat intake of healthy infants should not be restricted, and sources such as vegetable oils or soft vegan margarine should be included in the older infant's diet. Corn syrup should not be given to infants younger than one year old because of the risk of botulism, a form of food poisoning.

TYPICAL FEED FOR ONE DAY AT 12+ MONTHS

Breakfast- cereal or tahini on toast, breast or bottle-feed
Lunch- mixed vegetable dish with pulse base and a variety of
vegetables, rice pudding or fruit, and water or diluted fruit juice.

Snack. Baked apple and rice, soy yogurt
Dinner- breast or bottle feed

Throughout these early months of the infant's life, criticism may
be endured from friends, family or the medical establishment that
the diet is "reckless" or "experimental", but be assured that it is a
good healthy start to life. Many health professionals now
recognize that a vegan diet can be both nutritionally adequate
and health-promoting for both adults and children.

CHAPTER 8
FEEDING VEGAN INFANTS

A growing number of commercially- prepared baby foods are suitable for vegan infants, nevertheless, many parents opt to prepare their own baby foods, foods should be well washed, cooked thoroughly, and blended or mashed to an appropriate consistency. Home-prepared foods can be kept in the refrigerator for up to two days, or frozen in small quantities for later use.

- Infants need plenty of energy. Home-prepared cereals should be made as a thick porridge and not as a thin gruel. Add a little vegetable oil to the cooked grains to increase their calorie content and improve palatability by making them less glutinous as they cool.
- Use more soya bean oil or rapeseed (canola) oil, and less sunflower, safflower or corn oils. The former may encourage the production of fatty acids that are important for the development of the brain and vision.
- Do not allow infants to fill up with liquids before meal-times
- Spread breads with margarine fortified with D2 and B12 or with seed or nut butters to increase energy density.
- Low salt yeast extract is a good source of vitamins and minerals
- Well-cooked and mashed pulses provide energy and protein. Use black molasses to boost iron and calcium intakes
- Tofu prepared with calcium salt (usually calcium sulphate) contains more calcium than cow's milk, it is also rich in protein

- Make sure children have access to sunshine regularly and provide vitamin D2 supplements in winter.
- Use soya milk that is fortified with calcium, vitamin D2 and B12

PEANUTS AND ALLERGIES

Pediatricians do not recommend any sort of nut butters for children under 3 years, in families where there is a history if allergy, eczema or asthma, it is recommended that peanuts and peanut products be delayed until the child is at least 3 years old. Use peanuts and tree nuts of a suitable texture, but not before 4 months. Whole nuts are not recommended for the under-fives due to the risk of chocking. Peanuts are a good source of calcium and protein.

It is recommended that peanuts be avoided by pregnant or breast-feeding women if there is a history of allergies. It is finally suggested that women who are atopic 8(or where the father or any sibling has atopic disease) may wish to avoid peanuts in their diet to reduce the risk of their children developing peanut allergy, but this is simply precautionary as there has been no conclusive evidence.

CHAPTER 9
VEGAN TODDLERS AND PRESCHOOLERS

Toddlers and preschoolers, whether vegan or not, tend to eat less than most parents think they should, while nutrient needs are also relatively lower than during infancy, an adequate diet remains important to promote growth and development. These early years are also important for developing healthy eating patterns that can establish a foundation for a healthful adult diet. Young children have small stomachs, and too much high fiber food may make them feel full before they get all the calories they need. Foods such as avocados, nut and seed butters, dried fruit and soy products provide a concentrated source of calories. Dried fruits are also a concentrated source of energy and are attractive food for many children. Children from an early age should be encouraged to brush their teeth after eating dried fruits and other sweet foods to prevent tooth decay. If necessary, the fiber content of the diet can be reduced by giving some refined grain product, fruit juices and peeled fruits and vegetables. Eating more frequent meals, including nutritious snacks, can also help to ensure adequate energy intake.

GROWTH OF VEGAN CHILDREN

If your child's diet contains enough calories, normal growth and development can ne expected. Vegan children have been found to be slightly shorter and lighter in weight than average but appeared to be growing at a normal rate.

CHAPTER 10
INFORMATION ON KEY NUTRIENTS

PROTEIN

It is unnecessary to plan and complement amino acids precisely within each meal so long as children eat a variety of protein-rich foods each day. Sources of protein for vegan children include pulses (peas, beans, lentils, soy), grains (wheat, oats, rice, barley, buckwheat, millet, pasta, bread), nuts, meat substitutes and nut butters.

VITAMIN B12

B12 requirements for infants are 0.3mg per day for infants aged 0-6 months and 0.4ug for infants aged 6-12 months. Children from 1-10 years of age should consume 1ug increasing to 2ug per day. Because deficiency can have severe effects, and because natural plant sources of the vitamin (e.g. spirulina) are in serious doubts, it is important for vegan families to use and give their children fortified foods or supplements.

VITAMIN D

As sunlight during the winter is not strong enough in some countries to enable vitamin D synthesis in the skin, it is prudent to ensure a regular intake of vitamin D either from supplements or fortified foods all year round. Formula feeds contain sufficient vitamin D for infants, but breast milk may not supply adequate amounts, especially in northern countries in the winter. Some autumn-born babies who are solely breast fed throughout winter may develop a deficiency. Nutritional rickets is more likely to occur under these conditions in dark-skinned children. The vitamin D levels of breast milk can be increased by taking vitamin D supplements. It is recommended that vitamin drops containing vitamin A,C and D be used for all children from 6 months to 5 years of age.

Calcium

Calcium is an important nutrient for growing bones and teeth, given the importance of calcium intake during youth to lessening the future risk of osteoporosis, ensure calcium-rich foods in the diet. Good sources include fortified non-dairy milks and juices, calcium-set tofu, baked beans, and dark green leafy vegetables low in oxalic acid such as spring greens and kale. Calcium supplements are also an option. The reference nutrient intakes are 350-550mg per day for infants and children to the age of 10 years, 800mg per day for teenage girls, and 1000mg per day for teenage boys.

Iron

Iron deficiency anemia is the most common childhood nutritional problem, and is no more likely to occur in vegan than in non-vegan children. Good sources of iron include whole or enriched grain products, iron-fortified cereals, legumes, green leafy vegetables and dried fruit.

Zinc

Diet of vegan and non-vegan children often contain similar amounts of zinc, though zinc from plant food is less well absorbed as they contain phytate, which interferes with zinc absorption. Emphasizing foods that are good sources of zinc and protein such as pulses and nuts can increase the amount of zinc in the diet and promote absorption. Use of yeast-leavened bread and fermented soy products such as tempeh and miso can also improve zinc absorption. Zinc supplements may be needed for young vegan children whose diet is based on high-phytate cereals and legumes.

CHAPTER 11
THE TRANSITION TO A VEGAN DIET

Although today more and more children are vegan from birth, many older children also become vegan. There are many ways to make the transition from a non-vegan to a vegan diet. Some families gradually eliminate dairy products and eggs, while others make a more abrupt transition. Regardless of which approach you choose, be sure to explain what is going on, and why, in a way that your child can understand. Offer foods that look familiar at first. Peanut butter sandwiches seems to be universally popular, and many children like pasta or baked beans. Gradually introduce new foods. Watch your child's weight closely. Weight loss is likely at first, but if it continues, or the child seems to be growing less rapidly, add more concentrated calories and reduce the amount of fiber in the diet.

MANY VEGAN CHILDREN LIKE :

- Bagels with nut butter or hummus
- Bean burrito or tacos
- Fresh or dried fruit
- Mashed potatoes
- Oven-cooked chips
- Pancakes or waffles
- Pasta with tomato sauce
- Peanut butter and yeast extract sandwiches
- Pizza without cheese (or vegan cheese) topped with vegetables and pulses, tofu, or vegan meat
- Raw vegetables with dips
- Smoothies with soy milk
- Spaghetti with sauce
- Tofu/vegetarian dogs
- Veggie burgers

Chapter 12
Entertaining children and their friends
-The vegan party-

When dealing with non-vegan friends, it is worth making a note of the types of foods they will be likely to expect at parties. These foods may be slightly different from those that would be served to fellow vegans who may be eating a more wholefood-based diet children are notoriously undiplomatic in expressing their disapproval of food, especially at a birthday party or similar special gathering of friends. For example, avoid wholemeal breads if children are used to white flour. Carob in sweets or cakes is not a good idea if they have never eaten it before, as their taste buds are usually anticipating the sweet chocolate taste and are understandably disappointed. Buy in one of the many good quality vegan ice-creams on the market that should win over any non-vegan child. There is a recipe in the recipe section of the book with a good vegan sponge cake (chocolate is always popular) to round off the meal.

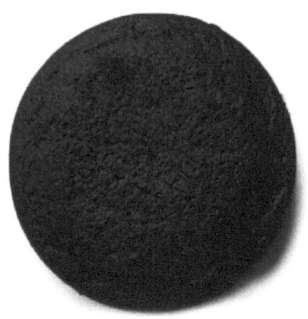

Chapter 13
Vegan school days

Whilst adults find it difficult to put up with criticism from relatives and friends, children may find it much harder, being more sensitive to criticism and peer pressure. Many simply want to "fit in" with the rest of the kids in the class, and not have to constantly defend their food and lifestyle. However, some kids actually rise to the occasion and enjoy being that little bit different! Other than at lunchtime, veganism is probably not going to be much of an issue at primary school. However, it is wise to prepare your children with sound information on veganism so they are able to stand firm against any comments coming their way.

In the case of secondary schools, animal rights as an issue is more and more popular with kids in their teens, and vegetarianism and veganism is becoming commonplace.

If you offer as much support, information on this subject as you would on any other about which you hold firm convictions, then this will give your kids a good grounding in veganism for the future. Children deserve to have information presented to them in a manner that takes account of their age, sensitivity and level of understanding. Honest answers and straight-talking will pay rich dividends at a later date. Children who are not fed an assortment of half-truths or deliberate misinformation will have little difficulty in making the connection between live animals and the food on their plate.

RECIPE

COOKBOOK

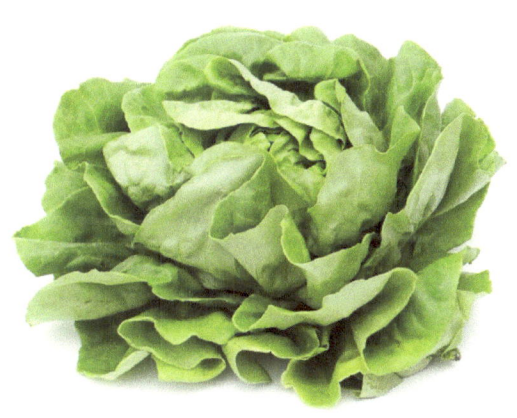

6-9 Months

Baby Muesli

Ingredients:
- 1 pear, peeled and chopped
- 5 dried apricots, simmered in a little water until soft
- 150 ml fortified soya milk
- 15 g oats

Procedure :

Place the oats and the soya milk in a saucepan and simmer for 3-4 minutes or until the mixture thickens, cool a little and place in a blender together with the cooked apricots and pear chunks. Blend until smooth and creamy.

Vegetable Puree

Ingredients:
- 1 large potato, peeled and chopped
- Florets removed from 1 broccoli stalk
- 1 courgette, sliced
- 2 or more tbsp soya milk

Procedure:

Steam or boil all the vegetables for around 10 minutes or until cooked. Cool a little and place in a blender together with the soya milk. Blend until smooth and creamy. Other vegetables can be used in this recipe instead of those listed.

Lentil Stew

Ingredients :

- 25 g dried red lentils
- 1 small potato, peeled and chopped
- ½ tsp tomato puree or tomato juice
- 1 small carrot, cubed

Procedure :

Place all the ingredients in a saucepan and just cover with water. Bring to the boil slowly and simmer until all the liquid is absorbed and the vegetables are softened. Cool a little and blend until smooth and creamy.

Baby's First Casserole

Ingredients :

- 1 small onion, finely chopped
- 1 medium carrot, diced
- 1 medium potato, diced
- 75 g dried red lentils
- 1 tsp. mixed dried herbs
- 50 g of tinned peas or beans
- 400 ml vegetable stock
- 1-2 tbsp. vegetable oil for frying

Procedure:

Fry the onion in a little vegetable oil until tender. Add the remaining ingredients and place in a casserole dish with lid. Place in a preheated oven at 180C°, 350F° for approximately 1 hour or until cooked. Cool a little before blending.

9-12+ Months

Minestrone Soup

Ingredients:

- 1 small onion, finely chopped
- ½ clove garlic, crushed
- 1 medium potato
- 1 medium carrot
- ½ stick celery
- 50 g cabbage, finely chopped
- 50 g peas
- 1 small tin haricot beans
- 75 g dried pasta shapes
- Vegetable oil for frying
- 1 liter of vegetable stock

Procedure :

Fry the onion and garlic in the vegetable oil. Add the celery and fry for a little longer. Add the remaining ingredients except the pasta and simmer for 20 minutes. Now add the pasta and simmer for a further 10 minutes.

Tip: instead of adding the pasta you could wait for the minestrone to cool down and blend it to make a creamy vegetable soup and top it with bread crumbs.

Lentil Soup

Ingredients:

- 50 g dried red lentils
- 1 small carrot, diced
- 280 ml soy milk
- 280 ml vegetable stock
- ½ tsp mixed herbs
- Seasoning: very little depending on age

Procedure:

Place all ingredients in a pan and simmer for 45 minutes. Allow to cool a little and then blend.

Bean Stew

Ingredients:

- 75 g dried peas and beans, soaked overnight
- 1 tbsp dried lentils
- 1 carrot, diced
- 1 small parnship, diced
- 1 small onion, finely chopped
- 15 g plain flour
- 1tbsp tomato puree
- ½ tsp mixed herbs
- ½ liter vegetable stock
- Vegetable oil for frying

Fry the onion lightly then add remaining ingredients except flour, bring to boil and simmer for 1 hour. Add tbsp of cold water to the flour and mix into paste. Add this to stew and cook for a few more minutes. Puree in a blender or, if child is older, serve as it is.

PASTA AND TOMATO SAUCE

Ingredients:
- 350 g jar pasta sauce
- 450 g firm plain tofu
- 3 tbsp soy sauce
- 2-3 adult portions of small dried pasta shells, bows or twists
- Boiling water to cook pasta

Procedure:
Cut the tofu into small cubes, cover in soy sauce and marinade for 30 minutes. In the meantime bring a large pan of water to the boil and place the pasta in the boiling water. Simmer until tender for approximately 10 minutes, wholemeal pasta will often take slightly longer. While the pasta is cooking, heat the pasta sauce in another pan together with the cubes of tofu. When the pasta has finished cooking, drain and add to the sauce along with the lightly fried vegetables (optional). Mix thoroughly and serve. This should make enough for around 1-2 adults depending on appetites.

Shepherd's Pie

Ingredients:

- 750g potatos, peeled,chopped
- 25g-50g vegan margarine
- 50ml or more soy milk
- ½ onion, finely chopped
- 150 ml vegetable stock
- Vegetable oil for frying
- 1 stick celery chopped
- 1 medium carrot diced
- 75g dried red lentils (cooked in water till tender)
- 1x400g tinned tomatoes

Procedure:

Steam the potatoes until soft and tender. Place in a separate bowl and add the margarine. Mash thoroughly adding the soy milk until the potato is smooth and creamy. Place aside. Heat the vegetable oil in frying pan and add the onions and celery. Fry until tender. Add the carrot, chopped tomatoes and 150ml vegetable stock. Simmer for 20 minutes, or until lentils are cooked and liquid is absorbed. Place in casserole dish and spread the creamed potato on top.

Heat in the oven at 180°, 350F for 15-20 minutes until potato is browned on top.

Vegetable Pasties

Ingredients:

- 100 g dried brown lentils
- 275 ml water for cooking lentils
- 3 medium carrots, diced
- 1 stick celery, finely chopped
- 220 g potatoes, diced
- 150 g peas, tinned or fresh
- 2 tsp yeast extract
- 2 tbsp. tomato puree
- ½ tsp mixed herbs
- Salt and pepper to taste (optional)
- 450 g short crust pastry (homemade or frozen)
- Soy milk to glaze

Procedure:

Wash lentils and boil water with celery for approximately 40 minutes until tender. Drain well. Steam or boil peas, carrots and potatoes until tender. Place all ingredients in a bowl and mix. Allow to cool. Roll out pastry and cut out rounds to make pasties. Make very small pasties so the child can easily hold them. Place a spoonful of filling in the middle of the pastry and moisten the edges with soy milk. Bring edges up together and press firmly to seal. Brush with coy milk to glaze and poke holes with a fork to allow hot air to escape whilst baking. Bake for 15-20 minutes at 200c°, 400F. Remove from oven when brown on top and allow to cool. They may be served hot or cold.

Fruit Tofu Dessert

Ingredients:
- 75 g mixed dried fruit
- 75 g silken tofu
- 50 g live soy yogurt

Procedure:
Gently cook dried fruit in a little water until soft and tender. Cool a little and blend with the yogurt and silken tofu until smooth and creamy.

Milky Fruit Jelly

Ingredients:
- 1 heaped tsp agar agar
- 250 ml pineapple or other sweet juice
- 250 ml concentrated fortified soy milk

Procedure:
Heat the soy milk and pineapple juice. Add agar agar and boil for 2-3 minutes. Place in mould and allow to set in the fridge.

Plain Fruit Jelly

Ingredients:
- 500-700 ml sweeten fruit juice, e.g. pineapple and mango
- 2 heaped tsp agar agar powder

Procedure:
Heat fruit juice until boiling. Add agar agar and allow to cook for 2-3 minutes. Pour into jelly mould and allow to set in fridge overnight. Serve with soy cream.

BIRTHDAY CAKES

These two recipes can either be made as described or the cake recipes can be used as a basic for creative birthday cake making e.g. bake in square cake tins, cut into blocks and cover with colored icing to make cars or trains. Add vegan chocolate biscuits for wheels, liquorice for bumpers, whizzers for door handles, etc. alternatively, bake in a round cake tin and decorate with colored icing to make a clown's face. Cakes can be imaginative and exciting as any non-vegan counterpart.

PLAIN SPONGE CAKE

Ingredients:
- 250 g self-raising wholemeal flour, sieved
- 75-100 g raw cane sugar
- 125 g margarine
- 3 tsp baking powder
- 275 ml vanilla soy dessert or custard
- ¼ tsp almond essence and/or vanilla essence
- Pinch of salt
- Soy milk

Procedure :
Over a low heat dissolve the margarine and sugar. Allow to cool. In a separate bowl mix together the dry ingredients. Add the margarine mixture to the dry ingredients and mix wee. Add the soya dessert or custard and essence. A soft dropping consistency is required so add extra soy milk if needed. Place in two square baking tins and bake for 25-30 minutes at 180C° or until cooked. Remove from oven and let cool completely. Sandwich with jam or butter icing made with vegan margarine and icing sugar.

CHOCOLATE CAKE

Ingredients :

- 200 g self-raising wholemeal flour
- 2 heaped tsp baking powder
- 25 g cocoa
- 75 g barbados sugar
- 100ml vegetable oil
- 550ml-700ml cold water
- 1 bar dark chocolate
- 1 pack of dairy free chocolate beans (40g)

Procedure :

Place all ingredients in food processor. Mix thoroughly for a few seconds. Place mixture in greased tin and bake for 30 minutes at 180C° in two round cake tins. Remove from the oven and allow to cool a little before removing. Melt bar of chocolate in a double bowl and spread on top of bake. Allow to set overnight and cut next day for best results. Mix icing sugar with a little hot water to soft consistency. Ice the top of the cake and place chocolate beans around the edges of the cake.

BUTTER ICING

Ingredients :

- 75g margarine
- 100g icing sugar
- 1 tsp vanilla essence

Procedure:

Beat the margarine and icing sugar until creamy. Add flavoring and beat again. Use as a filling for sponge cakes or for icing birthday cakes or cupcakes.

GROW GREEN

THE HEALTHY LIFESTYLE FOR YOU AND YOUR FAMILY
MAKE THE RIGHT CHOICES

FEDERICA LIPPI

www.ingramcontent.com/pod-product-compliance
Lightning Source LLC
Chambersburg PA
CBHW050822290526
45792CB00001B/222